The Complete Mediterranean Diet for Beginners

CHARLIE MASON

© Copyright 2017 by Charlie Mason - All rights reserved.

The follow Book is reproduced below with the goal of providing information that is as accurate and reliable as possible. Regardless, purchasing this eBook can be seen as consent to the fact that both the publisher and the author of this book are in no way experts on the topics discussed within and that any recommendations or suggestions that are made herein are for entertainment purposes only. Professionals should be consulted as needed prior to undertaking any of the action endorsed herein.

This declaration is deemed fair and valid by both the American Bar Association and the Committee of Publishers Association and is legally binding throughout the United States.

Furthermore, the transmission, duplication or reproduction of any of the following work including specific information will be considered an illegal act irrespective of if it is done electronically or in print. This extends to creating a secondary or tertiary copy of the work or a recorded copy and is only allowed with express written consent from the Publisher. All additional rights reserved.

The information in the following pages is broadly considered to be a truthful and accurate account of facts and as such any inattention, use or misuse of the information in question by the reader will render any resulting actions solely under their purview. There are no scenarios in which the publisher or the original author of this work can be in any fashion deemed liable for any hardship or damages that may befall them after undertaking information described herein.

Additionally, the information in the following pages is intended only for informational purposes and should thus be thought of as universal. As befitting its nature, it is presented without assurance regarding its prolonged validity or interim quality. Trademarks that are mentioned are done without written consent and can in no way be considered an endorsement from the trademark holder.

CONTENTS

1	The Characteristics of the Mediterranean Diet	Pg 4
2	Why Choose the Mediterranean Diet	Pg 7
3	A Brief History of the Mediterranean Diet	Pg 10
4	The Mediterranean Diet Pyramid	Pg 13
5	Tips to Supercharge Weight Loss	Pg 15
6	10 TOP MEDITERRANEAN RECIPES	Pg 18

CHAPTER 1: THE CHARACTERISTICS OF THE MEDITERRANEAN DIET

The Mediterranean diet doesn't incorporate anything fancy or complicated into its eating habits, instead focusing on the basics of eating healthy with a dash of olive oil and a glass or two of red wine added in for flavor. Broadly speaking it features as its chief components the traditional foods of the countries surrounding the Mediterranean Sea.

The diet includes plenty of healthy whole grains, fish, vegetables and fruits, while limiting unhealthy fats and processed foods. While these can all be said to be part of many healthy diets, there are variations in the Mediterranean Diet that can especially make a difference to those who are dealing with an increased risk of heart disease.

Crucial components

In general, the Mediterranean Diet emphasizes the regular consumption of plant-based foods including nuts, legumes, whole grains, vegetables and fruits. It also recommends switching out butter for other types of healthy fats such as canola or olive oil. Likewise, it recommends making a habit or replacing herbs and spices for flavoring foods rather than salt. As a rule, you should only eat red meat a few times each month, while also eating fish and poultry each at least twice per week.

When it comes to grains, nuts, vegetables and fruits, the number of servings you should aim for in a given day should reach Grecian levels. Greeks tend to eat only small amounts of red meat while consuming as many as nine servings of vegetables and fruits each day. Grains in this region tend to be of the whole grain variety and rarely contain any trans fats. The biggest difference with that region's dietary habits and the standard Western Diet is that they use olive oil for dipping bread in rather than margarine or butter, both of which contain saturated and trans fats. Another Mediterranean Diet alternative to butter for dipping is tahini sauce.

In general, you are going to want to strive for between seven and ten servings of fruits and vegetables per day. You are going to want to aim for high-quality whole grain bread and cereal and work more pasta and whole grain rice into your diet. These foods are rich in antioxidants and can benefit your body in a wide variety of different ways.

Nuts are another common part of the Mediterranean Diet. Nuts are comprised of about 80 percent healthy fats which makes them a great post-workout snack. They are extremely high in calories, however, so a little is going to go a long way. In generally, you are going to want to stick to a handful or two each day, and avoid anything that is heavily salted or honey-roasted.

When it comes to dealing with fat, the Mediterranean Diet doesn't focus on limiting total fat consumption and instead focuses on substituting good fats for bad fats. As such, the Mediterranean Diet discourages the consumption of hydrogenated oils which contain trans fats along with saturated fats, both of which are known to actively contribute to heart disease.

The Mediterranean Diet is also known for its heavy use of olive oil as its primary fat source. Olive oil provides monosaturated fat, which is a type of fat that is known to reduce bad cholesterol levels when it is used in place of more traditional trans or saturated fats. Virgin and extra virgin olive oils are often recommended as they are the least processed forms of the substance which means that they contain more of the beneficial plant compounds that generate the antioxidant effects that make the Mediterranean Diet so effective.

Additionally, polyunsaturated fats and monounsaturated fats, like those found in nuts and canola oil, contains a beneficial version of the omega-3 fatty acid known as linolenic acid. This fatty acid is known to lower triglycerides and decrease blood clotting and is generally associated with a decrease risk for heart attack. Likewise, fatty fish including salmon, tuna, albacore, sardines, herring, lake trout and mackerel are all known to be great sources of omega-3 fatty acids and the heavy consumption of fish is believed to be one of the things that makes the diet so effective overall. It should go without saying that you are going to want to cook the fish in the healthiest manner possible, no frying allowed.

Finally, while wine isn't considered a mandatory part of the diet, regular, and moderate, consumption of alcohol is known to be beneficial for a number of reasons. The average Mediterranean Diet tends to include about five ounces of wine per day for women and 10 ounces for men under the age of 65. If you have a family or personal history with alcohol abuse or liver or heart disease then it is strongly encouraged that you leave wine off of the menu.

CHAPTER 2: WHY CHOOSE THE MEDITERRANEAN DIET

Low in sugar and processed foods: As the diet is primarily made up of ingredients that are as close to nature as possible, this means that the foods you are going to be eating on the Mediterranean Diet will naturally be low in sugar, GMOs and other unnatural ingredients that are known to cause so much havoc within the human body when they are consumed on a regular basis.

Beyond plant-based foods, the Mediterranean Diet promotes the consumption of only a small amount of heavier meals and meats in general, instead favoring lighter and healthier options. This then naturally leads to weight loss and helps to improve omega-3 fatty acid intake, heart health and cholesterol.

Promotes healthy weight loss: When it comes to losing weight without feeling hungry, the Mediterranean Diet is a great way to go about doing so. The diet has the benefit of being both healthy and sustainable in the long-term meaning it is not so much a temporary fix, but a permanent lifestyle change. The focus on high quality proteins means that the diet can help keep you feeling full for longer, despite consuming fewer calories overall while also including additional benefits in the form of omega-3s and probiotics.

Furthermore, dairy, fish and red meat that is grass-fed contain high amounts of other types of healthy fatty acids that the body needs to help you feel full, control blood sugar, increase your overall energy level, improve your mood and moderate weight gain. If you are looking for a vegetarian or vegan option the diet still provides lots of protein options in the forms of whole grains and legumes.

Heart healthy choices: Studies show that sticking to the Mediterranean Diet, especially omega-3 rich foods and those high in monosaturated fats, is known to decrease mortality rate significantly, especially when it comes to issues related to heart disease. This is due to the linolenic acid found in olive oil which has been linked to decreasing the risk of cardiac death by as much as 30 percent and the risk of sudden death due to a cardiac event by as much as 45 percent.

What's more, research also shows that if the blood pressure of those who consume sunflower oil is compared to that of those who are consuming primarily extra-virgin olive oil, those who regularly consume the olive oil are going to have significantly lower results. It is also known to be beneficial when it comes to decreasing the effects of hypertension as it causes the body to generate more nitric acid which serves to counteract the process. Likewise, it also promotes oxidation while improving endothelial function which serves to counteract the condition.

Cancer fighting: The Mediterranean Diet is known to help combat the growth of a variety of cancer cells due to the way in which it provides the body with a measured amount of omega-3 and omega-6 fatty acids along with high amounts of polyphenols, antioxidants and fiber. As plant-based foods are a cornerstone of the Mediterranean Diet, then it can be said that eating in this way protects the very DNA from damage by decreasing the chances of cell mutation and inflammation which, in turn, helps to decrease the growth of tumors. There are also studies that show that olive oil could very well prove to be a natural cure for bowel and colon cancer. It has been shown to decrease the development of cancer cells in these regions as it lowers inflammation while also decreasing the rate of oxidative stress the body is under.

Helps get diabetes under control: The Mediterranean Diet is known to provide relief for diseases that are based around chronic inflammation such as type 2 diabetes and metabolic syndrome. One of the reasons that this is the case is the fact that the diet helps to control the excess production of insulin that is common in these issues. By regulating blood sugar levels through a balance of whole foods containing carbohydrates that are low in sugar, quality proteins and healthy fatty acids, the diet allows the body to burn fat more efficiently while maintaining more energy in the process.

Enhances cognitive processes: Recent research suggests that the Mediterranean Diet may prove to be a natural cure for Alzheimer's disease as well as dementia. These types of cognitive disorders are known to occur when the brain isn't receiving enough dopamine. Luckily, healthy fats such as that found in nuts and olive oil, when combined with the anti-inflammatory power of fruits and vegetables are known to fight off this type of cognitive decline. This occurs because the diet helps to counter the effectives that free radicals, toxicity and inflammation can have on the brain after a prolonged period of time.

CHAPTER 3: A BRIEF HISTORY OF THE MEDITERRANEAN DIET

The first version of the Mediterranean Diet was theorized in the 1970s by Ancel Keys, a biologist from America and his wife Margaret Keys a chemist and his writer and collaborator. However, it failed to gain widespread acceptance until it was reintroduced in 1993 by the European Office of the World Health Organization and the Harvard School of Public Health at a conference in Cambridge Massachusetts. Based on the dietary traditions of Greece, Crete and Southern Italy from around 1960, the original study found that rates in this area when it came to chronic diseases were some of the lowest in the entire world. Likewise, the life expectancy of the average adult in this area was among the longest in the world, despite the fact that many of the people in the region didn't have access to reliable healthcare.

The key to this longevity, the scientists who introduced it argued, was that the diet had resisted what at the time was approximately 50 years of efforts to modernize food that had been taking place at the time in many industrialized countries. These trends in modernization tended to lead towards a diet that contained more beef and other animal products, while at the same time overall fewer fruits and vegetables and a much higher concentration of processed foods.

On the contrary, the diet of the region in question continued to consist mainly of vegetables, fruits, whole grains and fish, along with plenty of olive oil and wine, of course. Other vital elements of the Mediterranean Diet, the study insisted included plenty of daily exercise along with the practice of eating meals in groups and taking the time to more fully appreciate food before consuming it. This, in turn, naturally leads to a more leisurely meal pace which means that food has more time to pass through the body before the meal is complete, leading to smaller portion sizes as well.

While it may seem odd today, with millionaires paying untold sums for third world delicacies and celebrities subsisting on water, cayenne pepper and lemon juice, one of the biggest reasons that the Mediterranean Diet failed to catch on initially was that it was seen as a diet for the poor. In fact, when Keys did the initial study, Portugal was also listed as one of the main regional contributors to the diet. However, the leader of Portugal didn't want his country to be listed among the countries polled for this diet of the poor so the country was stricken from the dietary record.

Soon after it began to gain popularity in the mainstream, a number of companies from the agriculture and food sectors in Barcelona got together to essentially promote their brand while telling the people that abandoning the traditional eating habits of their people would do them little good in the long run. This group became the Association for the Advancement of the Mediterranean Diet in late 1995 with the stated mission of encouraging the consumption of traditional Mediterranean products for the health benefits of all.

This group then joined with a number of other similarly themed organizations to form the Mediterranean Diet Foundation in 1996. The mission of the foundation is to promote keen insight into the benefits surrounding the Mediterranean Diet when it comes to gastronomical, cultural, historical and health aspects. Furthermore, the foundation aims to disseminate scientific findings regarding the diet and the ways it can benefit the health of people around the world.

Since its inception, the FDM has been involved in a wide variety of activities, starting with the spreading of a wide variety of research through the use of biennial conferences that take place during large international food exhibitions. At the Alimentaria conference in 1996, the Barcelona Declaration on the Mediterranean Diet was signed by the FDM, the Barcelona City Countil, Fish and Food, the Spanish Ministry of Agriculture and the Food and Agriculture Organization. Later that same year the Grande Covian award was created to recognize professionals who had contributed greatly to the study of the Mediterranean Diet.

The FDM has also been granting honorary diplomas since the start of the 00s to individuals who have proven that they excel when it comes to their contributions in the social and cultural sphere when it comes to promoting the Mediterranean Diet and Mediterranean culture. Individuals recognized in this way so far include Juan Antonio Corbalán, Bigas Luna, Joan Manuel Serrat, Georges Moustaki and the great Ferran Adrià. These awards are given out during each biennial conference at the same time as the Grande Covian. The group has also formed a partnership with the FOOD Program which is working to influence dietary changes in the workplace and is specifically targeting habits and lifestyles that are directly known to lead to obesity.

CHAPTER 4: THE MEDITERRANEAN DIET PYRAMID

The Mediterranean Diet Pyramid was developed and released at the same time as the Mediterranean Diet was being reintroduced to the public in the 1990s. It sums up the way that the diet suggests that followers break up their eating patterns, making it easier to determine the types of foods you should eat each day. The pyramid is, unsurprisingly, also closely tied to areas of olive oil cultivation in the Mediterranean. The Mediterranean Diet Pyramid is broken into monthly, weekly and daily units, but does not list serving sizes other than to note to keep meals reasonably sized.

The original Mediterranean Diet Pyramid was created using then current nutritional research as a means of representing a well-rounded Mediterranean diet. It recommended potatoes, grains, bulgur, polenta, couscous, rice, pasta and breads with every meal. Fruits, vegetables and olive oil were recommended on a daily basis along with smaller amounts of yogurt and cheese. It recommended fish and poultry a few times a week and sweets and red meat sparingly, only a few times a month. Red wine was also recommended in moderation. A new layer added to the bottom of the pyramid to account for the need for daily exercise was also added in 2000 as fears about a nationwide obesity epidemic first started materializing. While the original graph was nothing but simple words, the pyramid was soon updated with various graphics to ensure that the foods at each level were clear.

While the graphics were updated over the years, the science underlying the Mediterranean Diet Pyramid remained the same for the next fifteen years. For that year's Mediterranean Diet Conference, however, Harvard scientists decided to review the pyramid in light of nutritional findings that had come to light in the previous decade and a half of academic research. One of the biggest changes to the pyramid at this time was the addition of spices and herbs as a replacement for salt when it comes to maximizing taste. It also serves to make the pyramid more accurate as these spices and herbs contribute significantly to the national identities of many of the dishes that are a core of the Mediterranean Diet.

Additionally, the scientists changed the placement of fish on the pyramid and also added shellfish to the list, noting that the increase to at least twice a week would better serve to emphasize the benefits that are gained when omega-6 fatty acids and omega-3 fatty acids are in balance with one another. An advisory board was also convened which came to a consensus on several other aspects of the Mediterranean Diet Pyramid as well. These changes primarily centered around gathering olive oil, olives, seeds, legumes, nuts, grains, vegetables into a single group to make it clear that they are all on the same page when it comes to health benefits. The goal with this change was to also draw extra attention to the key role that these foods should play in the health-promoting pattern of the diet and also to put all of these items onto equal footing.

This update to the terms of the pyramid prompted a visual update in 2009 with the help of artist George Middleton. He created an entirely new graphic to represent the pyramid that reflects the current most effective grouping of foods according to the experts. The pyramid now shows physical activity, eating with others and enjoying your meals at the bottom, followed by a very large space for fruits, vegetables, whole grains, olive oil, nuts, beans, legumes, seeds, spice and herbs to be consumed with every meal. Above that is fish and other seafood which should be consumed at least twice each week. Next is yogurt, cheese, eggs and poultry which can be consumed multiple times in a week. At the top is still sweets and red meat which should be consumed just a few times each month. Finally, it recommends drinking lots of water and wine in moderation.

CHAPTER 5: TIPS TO SUPERCHARGE WEIGHT LOSS

Never skip a meal: While it may seem to make sense that skipping the occasional meal should promote weight loss, after all you are eating fewer calories in a given day, the fact is the opposite is true. This is because your body gets into a habit of taking in and burning calories throughout the day based on your average eating patterns and missing a meal gums up the works. Rather than taking in and burning calories as anticipated, your body now needs to stretch what was already available further than it was planning to which means it will have to play catchup later on. This, in turn, means that skipping that meal will likely cause you to hold onto more weight that day, not less as your body will try and hold onto everything it can until it knows just what is going on.

You should always start your day off with a healthy and nutritious breakfast as this will kick your metabolism into gear at the start of the day, keeping it in the habit of not holding onto any additional fat throughout the day. Ideally you will want to split your day up into three moderate meals and then three light snacks so that you are eating about every three hours. This will ensure that once your metabolism gets going in the morning, it won't stop, burning more calories overall throughout the day than you would otherwise. It is important to watch what you consume with this strategy, however, as choosing unhealthy snacks will negate any work that you are doing by sticking to the Mediterranean Diet.

Lift weights: Your body will naturally burn more fat if it is full of muscle instead of just more fat. As such, the more muscle you build on the regular, the more calories your body will burn every day, even while at rest. Muscle burns fat which means that your metabolism will also increase if your overall muscle mass is higher. This means that if you start weight training then you will likely see the fat melt off faster than you might think as you are now burning fat while exercising, and then burning more fat than ever before, even while at rest.

In order to take things up to the next level, you will also want to add in a mixture of high intensity workouts to your regular exercise routine. These high intensity workouts are usually 30 minutes or less and include a quick burst of cardio in addition to the weights. Adding it in at random intervals will make it hard for your body to anticipate the extra effort required which will cause your metabolism to go into overdrive as a result. It is important to not overdo it, however, as high intensity workouts can easily lead to strain.

Drink the right caffeinated beverages: When consumed without any additives, both coffee and tea can help you jump-start your metabolism. The one thing you should never drink, however, is soda, even if it doesn't have any calories. The wide variety of artificial ingredients in diet sodas can have a wide variety of unpredictable effects on the body, including causing you to hold onto fat that you otherwise would have already ditched. Rather than stick with artificial stuff, you should focus on herbal teas such as Skinny Teatox which can really help you knock off the extra pounds. This is the case because the herbs in these teas are known to improve the rate at which your body metabolizes food while also decreasing the response that fat cells have to sugar. Finally, they are also known to improve the way that fat cells react to insulin which, in turn, helps to aid in digestion and increase the overall functionality of the metabolism.

When it comes to coffee, you should drink it black as the antioxidant catechins it contains have been proven to add a boost to the metabolic system. What's more, if you drink a double shot of espresso before you exercise you are likely to burn as many as 20 percent more calories than you would otherwise. You will see some benefit if you drink your cup of joe directly after exercising as well, though the effects will be lessened.

Embrace the cold: The more energy that your body requires in order to normalize its temperature, the higher your metabolism will remain overall. Essentially, what this means is that if you exercise in the cold your body will be required to burn more energy just to reach its core required temperature. The colder it is when you exercise the greater the amount of bad fat that you will burn in the interim. You can also increase your metabolism in this fashion by drinking lots of ice water and regularly taking ice-cold showers.

Drink more water: Water is a crucial element of life and, like most aspects of the way the body functions, the metabolism cannot work properly without enough water. The average person is more dehydrated than they should be more than 70 percent of the time. Don't think you are in that majority? Ask yourself if you are thirsty right now. If the answer is yes then you are already dehydrated. Ideally you are going to want to aim to drink a gallon of water each day. This is a gallon of water a day, pure, water with additives doesn't count. The more you can manage in a day, the more smoothly your metabolism will run at all times and the more weight you will lose every day.

Eat more spicy foods: The capsaicin spice, what causes the heat in most spicy foods is also known to increase your metabolism. This is due to the fact that eating it causes the body's internal temperature to increase which means that it needs to work harder to remain parity with the outside temperature. As a general rule, if a meal is hot enough to make you start to sweat, then it is going to be hot enough to increase your metabolism as well.

CHAPTER 6: 10 TOP MEDITERRANEAN RECIPES

1: Grecian Chicken Pasta

This recipe needs 15 minutes to prepare, 15 minutes to cook and will make 6 servings.

- Protein: 32.6 grams
- Carbs: 70 grams
- Fats: 11.4 grams
- Calories: 488

What to Use

- Olive oil (1 T)
- Red onion (.5 c chopped)
- Linguine (16 oz.)
- Pepper (as desired)
- Salt (as desired)
- Lemons (2 wedged)
- Oregano (2 tsp. dried)
- Lemon juice (2 T)
- Parsley (3 T chopped)
- Feta cheese (.5 c crumbled)
- Tomato (1 chopped)
- Marinated artichoke hearts (14 oz. chopped, drained)
- Chicken breast (1 lb. cubed)
- Garlic (2 cloves crushed)

What to Do

- Fill a large pot with water and a pinch of salt before placing it on the stove on top of a burner that has been turned to a high heat. Once the water boils, add in the pasta and let it cook until it is still firm but just starting to become tender, which should take approximately 8 minutes.
- Add the olive oil to a skillet before placing it on top of a burner turned to a high/medium heat. Place the garlic and onion into the

skillet and let it cook for approximately 2 minutes until it begins to be fragrant.
- Mix in the chicken and stir regularly until the chicken ceases to be pink and all of its juices are clear, this should take approximately 5 minutes. The chicken should end up with an internal temperature of 165F.
- Turn the burner to a low/medium heat before adding in the pasta, oregano, lemon juice, parsley, feta cheese, tomato and artichoke hearts. Let the results cook while stirring for roughly 2 minutes.
- Remove the skillet from the burner, season as desired and garnish using the lemon prior to serving.

2: Feta and Spinach Bake

This recipe needs 10 minutes to prepare, 12 minutes to cook and will make 6 servings.

- Protein: 11.6 grams
- Carbs: 41.6 grams
- Fats: 17.1 grams
- Calories: 350

What to Use

- Pepper (as desired)
- Salt (as desired)
- Extra virgin olive oil (2 T)
- Parmesan cheese (2 T)
- Feta cheese (.5 c crumbled)
- Mushrooms (4 sliced)
- Spinach (1 bunch chopped, rinsed)
- Roma tomatoes (2 chopped)
- Whole wheat pita (6, 6 in.)
- Sun-dried tomato peso (6 oz.)

What to Do

- Ensure your oven is heated to 350F.

- Top one side of each pita using the sun-dried tomato peso before placing them face-up on a baking sheet. Top with mushrooms, spinach and tomatoes before adding the parmesan and feta cheese and topping with olive oil and seasoning as desired.
- Place the baking sheet in the oven and let the pita bake until they are crisp which should take approximately 10 minutes.
- Quarter the pita prior to serving.

3: White Beans, Tomatoes and Greek Pasta

This recipe needs 10 minutes to prepare, 15 minutes to cook and will make 4 servings.

- Protein: 23.4 grams
- Carbs: 79 grams
- Fats: 5.9 grams
- Calories: 460

What to Use

- Pepper (as desired)
- Salt (as desired)
- Feta cheese (.5 c crumbled)
- Penne pasta (8 oz.)
- Spinach (10 oz. chopped, washed)
- Cannellini beans (19 oz. rinsed, drained)
- Italian style tomatoes (14.5 oz. diced)

What to Do

- Fill a large pot with water and a pinch of salt before placing it on the stove on top of a burner that has been turned to a high heat. Once the water boils, add in the pasta and let it cook until it is just starting to become tender which should take about 8 minutes.
- While the pasta is cooking, add the olive oil to a skillet before placing it on top of a burner turned to a high/medium heat. Add in the beans and the tomatoes and let everything boil. After this occurs, reduce the heat to low/medium and let everything simmer for 10 minutes.
- Add in the spinach and let it cook for 2 minutes or until it starts to wilt, stirring regularly.

- Plate pasta and top with sauce and crumbled feta prior to serving.

4: Cannellini Beans and Pasta

This recipe needs 5 minutes to prepare, 20 minutes to cook and will make 8 servings.

- Protein: 8.2 grams
- Carbs: 30.5 grams
- Fats: 4.2 grams
- Calories: 185

What to Use

- Pepper (as desired)
- Salt (as desired)
- Seashell pasta (.25 lbs.)
- Basil (1 tsp.)
- Parsley (.25 c)
- Cannellini beans (15 oz.)
- Low-sodium chicken broth (3 c)
- Tomatoes (14.5 oz. stewed)
- Garlic (3 cloves minced)
- Onion (1 c chopped)
- Extra virgin olive oil (2 T)

What to Do

- Add the oil to a Dutch oven that is at least 4 quarts before placing it on top of a medium heat. After it warms, add in the garlic and onions and let them cook for approximately 5 minutes or until the onion is nice and tender.
- Mix in the basil, parsley, chicken broth, tomatoes and cannellini beans and season as desired before turning the heat to high and letting everything boil. Let everything boil for 60 seconds and then turn the heat to low/medium and let everything simmer for 10 minutes with the Dutch oven covered.
- Mix in the pasta and let everything simmer for about 10 minutes

until the pasta is extremely tender.

5: Sicilian Spaghetti

This recipe needs 10 minutes to prepare, 5 minutes to cook and will make 8 servings.

- Protein: 12.4 grams
- Carbs: 53.6 grams
- Fats: 9.8 grams
- Calories: 355

What to Use

- Pepper (as desired)
- Salt (as desired)
- Extra virgin olive oil (2 T)
- Parmesan cheese (4 T grated)
- Parsley (1 c)
- Bread crumbs (1 c)
- Anchovy filets (2 oz. chopped)
- Garlic (3 cloves crushed)
- Olive oil (4 T)
- Spaghetti (1 lb.)

What to Do

- Fill a large pot with water and a pinch of salt before placing it on the stove on top of a burner that has been turned to a high heat. Once the water boils, add in the pasta and let it cook for approximately 8 minutes and has reach an al dente state. Drain the pasta and set aside.
- While the pasta cooks, add the olive oil to a skillet before placing it on top of a burner turned to a high/medium heat. Place the garlic and anchovies into the skillet and let them cook for approximately 2 minutes, stirring constantly.
- Add in the breadcrumbs before turning the heat off on the burner. Add in the parsley and season as desired before mixing

well.
- Toss the pasta and the sauce together and top with cheese prior to serving.

6: Broccoli and Cavatelli

This recipe needs 10 minutes to prepare, 20 minutes to cook and will make 12 servings.

- Protein: 10.2 grams
- Carbs: 47.6 grams
- Fats: 10.3 grams
- Calories: 317

What to Use

- Pepper (as desired)
- Salt (as desired)
- Extra virgin olive oil (.5 c)
- Parmesan cheese (2 T)
- Red pepper flakes (1 tsp.)
- Cavatelli pasta (1.5 lbs.)
- Garlic (3 cloves minced)
- Broccoli (3 heads florets)

What to Do

- Fill a large pot with water before adding in the broccoli and placing it on top of the stove over a burner turned to a high heat. Let the broccoli blanch for roughly 5 minutes before draining the broccoli and setting aside
- Refill the large pot with water and a pinch of salt before placing it on the stove on top of a burner that has been turned to a high heat. Once the water boils, add in the pasta and let it cook for approximately 8 minutes until it has reached an al dente state. Once it has finished cooking, drain it and add it to a large serving bowl.
- While the pasta is cooking, add the olive oil to a skillet before placing it on top of a burner turned to a high/medium heat. Place

the garlic into the skillet and let it sauté until it starts to turn a golden hue, take care to ensure it doesn't burn. Mix in the broccoli and let it cook for about 10 minutes, stirring occasionally, the broccoli should be slightly tender but still largely crisp.

• Toss the broccoli with the pasta and season well. Top with parmesan cheese prior to serving.

7: Shrimp and Penne

This recipe needs 10 minutes to prepare, 20 minutes to cook and will make 8 servings.

- Protein: 24.5 grams
- Carbs: 48.5 grams
- Fats: 8.5 grams
- Calories: 385

What to Use

- Pepper (as desired)
- Salt (as desired)
- Extra virgin olive oil (2 T)
- Parmesan cheese (1 c grated)
- Shrimp (1 lb. deveined, peeled)
- Tomatoes (29 oz. diced)
- White wine (.25 c)
- Garlic (1 T chopped)
- Red onion (.25 c)
- Olive oil (2 T)
- Penne pasta (16 oz.)

What to Do

• Fill a large pot with water and a pinch of salt before placing it on the stove on top of a burner that has been turned to a high heat. Once the water boils, add in the pasta and let it cook for about 8 minutes until it reaches an al dente state.

• Add the olive oil to a skillet before placing it on top of a burner turned to a high/medium heat. Place the garlic and onion into the skillet and cook until the onion begins to turn tender. Add in the wine along with the tomatoes and let everything cook for 10

minutes, stirring regularly.
- Add in the shrimp and let it cook for 5 minutes. Toss with the pasta and top with parmesan cheese prior to serving.

8: Mediterranean Falafel

This recipe needs 20 minutes to prepare, 20 minutes to cook and will make 4 servings.

- Protein: 11.4 grams
- Carbs: 39.3 grams
- Fats: 9.3 grams
- Calories: 281

What to Use

- Pepper (as desired)
- Extra virgin olive oil (2 T)
- All-purpose flour (1 T)
- Baking soda (.25 T)
- Salt (.25 tsp.)
- Coriander (.25 tsp. ground)
- Cumin (1 tsp. ground)
- Garlic (3 cloves minced)
- Parsley (.25 c chopped)
- Garbanzo beans (15 oz. drained, rinsed)
- Onion (.25 c chopped)

What to Do

- Place the chopped onion into a cheese cloth and squeeze it as hard as possible to remove any excess water.
- Add the baking soda, salt, coriander, cumin, garlic, parsley and garbanzo beans into your food processor and process until the

results are becoming pureed but are still somewhat coarse.
- In a mixing bowl, combine the results from the food processor along with the onion and mix well prior to adding in the egg along with the flour. Mix well and shape the results into patties.
- Ensure your oven is set to 400F
- While the oven is warming, add the olive oil to your oven-safe skillet and place it on top of the stove over a burner turner to a high/medium heat. Add the patties to the skillet and let them cook approximately 2.5 minutes per side or until they take on a golden-brown color.
- Remove the skillet from the stove and place it in the oven. Let the falafel cook approximately 10 minutes or until it is warm all the way through.
- Serve with pita bread and tzatziki and enjoy.

9: Flounder with capers, olives and tomatoes

This recipe needs 20 minutes to prepare, 20 minutes to cook and will make 4servings.

- Protein: 24.4 grams
- Carbs: 8.2 grams
- Fats: 15.4 grams
- Calories: 282

What to Use

- Pepper (as desired)
- Extra virgin olive oil (2 T)
- Basil (6 leaves torn)
- Flounder (1 lb. fillets)
- Parmesan cheese (3 T grated)
- Basil (6 leaves chopped)
- Lemon juice (1 tsp. fresh)
- Capers (.25 c)
- White wine (.25 c)
- Kalamata olives (24 chopped, pitted)
- Italian seasoning (1 pinch)
- Garlic (2 cloves chopped)
- Spanish onion (.5 chopped)
- Tomatoes (5 rinsed)

What to Do

- Ensure your oven is heated to 425F.
- Fill a saucepan with water and a pinch of salt before placing it on the stove on top of a burner that has been turned to a high heat. Once the water boils, add in the tomatoes before pulling them right back out again. Ensure you have a bowl of cold water ready to add them to. Once they are cool enough to handle, remove the skin prior to chopping.
- Add the olive oil to the skillet before placing the skillet on the stove on top of a burner set to a medium heat. Add in the onion and let it cook for about 5 minutes until it is tender. Add in the Italian seasoning, garlic and tomatoes and let everything cook about 6 minutes.
- Add in half of the basil, the lemon juice, capers, wine and olives before turning the heat down and mixing in the parmesan cheese. Let everything cook approximately 15 minutes and it has formed a thick sauce.
- Add the flounder to a baking dish before topping with sauce and basil leaves.
- Place the dish in the oven and let it cook about 10 minutes until the flesh of the fish can easily be flaked with a fork.

10: Costa Brava

This recipe needs 10 minutes to prepare, 25 minutes to cook and will make 10servings.

- Protein: 28.6 grams
- Carbs: 17.6 grams
- Fats: 6.1 grams
- Calories: 239

What to Use

- Pepper (as desired)
- Extra virgin olive oil (2 T)
- Red bell pepper (1 sliced thin)

- Water (2 T)
- Cornstarch (2 T)
- Salsa (.5 c)
- Black olives (2 c)
- Stewed tomatoes (14.5 oz.)
- Yellow onion (1 quartered)
- Garlic (2 cloves minced)
- Cinnamon (1 tsp)
- Cumin (1 tsp)
- Chicken breasts (5 halved)
- Pineapple chunks (20 oz.)

What to Do
- Drain the pineapple but keep the juice. Likely sprinkle salt on top.
- Add the oil to a pan before placing it on the stove on top of a burner turned to a high/medium heat. Add in the chicken before topping with cinnamon and cumin. Mix in the onion and garlic and let everything cook for about 5 minutes.
- Mix in the salsa, olives, tomatoes and pineapple juice. Cover the pan and reduce the heat to allow everything to simmer approximately 25 minutes.
- After the pan has finished simmering, combine the water and cornstarch and add it to the pan juices. Mix in the bell pepper and let the pan simmer until it forms a sauce. Mix in the pineapple chunks and let them simmer until they are warm.
- Top the chicken with the sauce prior to serving.

CONCLUSION

Thank for making it through to the end of this book, let's hope it was informative and able to provide you with all of the tools you need to achieve your goals whatever they may be.

The next step is to start using some of these great recipes in your own home.

Finally, if you found this book useful in any way, a review on Amazon is always appreciated!

Printed in Great Britain
by Amazon